COMPLETE GUIDE TO LIMB LENGTHENING SURGERY

Essential Handbook To Modern Techniques, Recovery, And Best Practices For Optimal Results

DR. BRUNO HORAN

Copyright © 2023 by Dr. Bruno Horan

All rights reserved. Except for brief quotations embodied in critical reviews and certain other noncommercial uses permitted by copyright law, no part of this publication may be reproduced, distributed, or transmitted in any form or by any means, Including photocopying, recording, or other electronic or mechanical methods, without the prior written permission of the publisher.

Disclaimer:

The information provided in this book, is intended for general informational purposes only and should not be considered as professional advice.

The author has made every effort to ensure the accuracy of the information presented. However, readers are advised to consult with a qualified healthcare professional before attempting any herbal remedies or making significant changes to their wellness routine. Individual health conditions vary, and what may be suitable for one person may not be appropriate for another.

It is important to note that the author is not in any endorsement deal, partnership, or affiliation with any organization, brand, or company mentioned in this book. Any references to specific products or services are based on the author's personal experience or general knowledge and do not imply an endorsement or promotion of those products or services

Contents

CHAPTER ONE 13

  UNDERSTANDING LIMB LENGTHENING SURGERY 13

    Definition And Goals Of Limb Lengthening 13

    Types Of Limb Length Discrepancies 14

    Benefits And Risks Of The Procedure 15

CHAPTER TWO 19

  PREPARING FOR LIMB LENGTHENING SURGERY .. 19

    Initial Consultation And Evaluations 19

    Psychological Preparation For Surgery 20

    Physical Preparation And Pre-Operative Instructions 20

    Anesthesia Options And Considerations 21

    Preparing Your Home And Support System 22

CHAPTER THREE 23

  RECOVERY PHASE AND REHABILITATION 23

    Immediate Post-Surgery Care 23

    Managing Pain And Discomfort 24

    Physical Therapy And Rehabilitation Exercises 25

    Nutritional Considerations For Recovery 26

Monitoring Progress And Adjusting Treatment Plans 27

CHAPTER FOUR 29

POTENTIAL COMPLICATIONS AND RISKS 29

Common Complications During And After Surgery 29

Long-Term Risks And Challenges 30

Strategies For Complication Prevention 31

Addressing The Psychological Impact Of Surgery 32

Patient Stories And Coping Strategies 32

CHAPTER FIVE 35

LIFE AFTER LIMB LENGTHENING SURGERY 35

Adjusting To New Limb Lengths 35

Physical And Psychological Adaptation 36

Returning To Daily Activities And Work 38

Follow-Up Care And Monitoring 39

Maintaining Long-term Bone Health 39

CHAPTER SIX 41

ALTERNATIVE TREATMENTS AND THERAPIES 41

Non-Surgical Options For Limb Length Discrepancies 41

Comparative Benefits And Drawbacks 43
Integrative Therapies For Rehabilitation 44
Case Studies And Patient Experiences 46
CHAPTER SEVEN 49
COMMON CONCERNS AND FAQS 49
Addressing Pain Management Concerns 50
Dealing With Length Discrepancy Correction 51
Managing External Fixator Or Device Discomfort. 52
CHAPTER EIGHT 55
LOOKING AHEAD: ADVANCES IN LIMB LENGTHENING 55
Innovations In Surgical Techniques 55
Future Prospects For Limb-Lengthening Technology 56
Research And Development In Bone Regeneration 58
Patient Advocacy And Support Networks 59
Recommendations For Further Reading And Resources 60

ABOUT THIS BOOK

Limb Lengthening Surgery: A Comprehensive Guide delves into a transformative realm of orthopedic surgery, offering invaluable insights into a procedure that significantly impacts quality of life.

This guide is an essential resource for patients, caregivers, and healthcare professionals seeking a deeper understanding of limb-lengthening surgery.

By exploring its history, surgical techniques, recovery phases, and future advancements, this book empowers readers with knowledge crucial to making informed decisions and achieving optimal outcomes.

At the core of this guide lies a thorough exploration of limb-lengthening surgery. It illuminates the procedure's definition, goals, and the diverse types of limb length discrepancies it addresses.

From eligibility criteria to meticulous descriptions of surgical processes, this section navigates readers through every stage of preparation and anesthesia considerations. Detailed insights into surgical techniques, bone regeneration, and post-operative care reinforce a comprehensive understanding essential for navigating this transformative journey.

Following surgery, the recovery phase unfolds crucial chapters focusing on immediate post-operative care, pain management strategies, and tailored rehabilitation exercises.

Nutritional guidance supports recovery while ongoing monitoring ensures adjustments align with progress. This section not only prepares individuals practically but also psychologically, nurturing resilience during a transformative rehabilitation process.

Navigating the complexities of limb-lengthening surgery entails awareness of potential complications and long-term risks. This section equips readers with preemptive strategies for complication prevention and addresses psychological impacts through patient stories and coping mechanisms. By candidly exploring challenges, this guide promotes proactive engagement with recovery hurdles, fostering informed decision-making and holistic patient care.

Beyond recovery, this guide illuminates life post-surgery, offering practical guidance on adjusting to new limb lengths and sustaining long-term bone health.

It facilitates a seamless return to daily activities while advocating for integrative therapies and lifestyle adjustments that support ongoing well-being.

Case studies and FAQs enrich this section, offering diverse perspectives and solutions to common concerns, and ensuring readers approach their new chapter with confidence and clarity.

Concluding with a visionary outlook, this guide explores prospects in limb-lengthening technology and bone regeneration. It celebrates ongoing research, innovations in surgical techniques, and the evolving landscape of patient advocacy and support networks. Recommendations for further reading and resources empower readers to stay informed and engaged with advancements shaping the future of limb-lengthening surgery.

Through its comprehensive scope and compassionate approach, Limb Lengthening Surgery: A Comprehensive Guide emerges as a beacon of knowledge and empowerment. It navigates the complexities of orthopedic surgery with clarity and empathy, ensuring readers embark on their journey towards enhanced mobility and quality of life fully informed and supported.

CHAPTER ONE

UNDERSTANDING LIMB LENGTHENING SURGERY

Limb lengthening surgery is a complex orthopedic procedure designed to increase the length of a bone or correct limb length discrepancies. It is typically performed to address conditions where a person has unequal limb lengths due to various factors such as congenital anomalies, growth plate injuries, or conditions like dwarfism.

Definition And Goals Of Limb Lengthening

The primary goal of limb lengthening surgery is to increase the length of a bone in the affected limb. This can improve the patient's overall limb symmetry, functionality, and often their quality of life.

The procedure involves carefully cutting the bone (osteotomy) and then gradually distracting it using an external or internal fixation device. Over time, new bone forms in the gap created by distraction, resulting in increased length.

Types Of Limb Length Discrepancies

Limb length discrepancies can be categorized into several types based on their causes and severity. They include congenital limb length differences present from birth, acquired discrepancies due to trauma or infection affecting bone growth, and functional discrepancies caused by joint contractures or muscle imbalances.

Patient Eligibility Criteria

Candidates for limb lengthening surgery typically include individuals who have significant limb length discrepancies that affect their daily functioning or cause discomfort.

The decision for surgery is often made after thorough evaluation by orthopedic surgeons who assess factors such as the patient's skeletal maturity, overall health, and realistic expectations regarding the procedure and recovery.

Benefits And Risks Of The Procedure

The benefits of limb lengthening surgery include improved limb symmetry, enhanced function, and psychological well-being for patients who may have experienced social or physical challenges due to their condition.

However, the procedure also carries risks such as infection at the surgical site, complications related to the fixation devices, nerve or blood vessel damage, and prolonged rehabilitation periods.

Overview of the Surgical Process

Preparation: Before surgery, the patient undergoes thorough medical evaluations and imaging scans to plan the procedure. The surgical team discusses the goals, risks, and expected outcomes with the patient.

Surgical Procedure: During the surgery, the orthopedic surgeon makes precise cuts in the bone (osteotomy) at the predetermined site. This is followed by the placement of an external or internal fixation device, which allows for controlled distraction of the bone segments.

Distraction Phase: Over several weeks to months, depending on the rate of new bone formation, the bone segments are gradually distracted (pulled apart) by adjusting the fixation device. This stimulates the growth of new bone tissue in the gap created.

Consolidation Phase: Once the desired length is achieved, the distraction phase is followed by a consolidation phase where the bone gradually hardens and becomes stronger.

During this period, physical therapy and rehabilitation play a crucial role in restoring strength, flexibility, and function to the limb.

Device Removal: In some cases, once the bone has fully healed and consolidated, the fixation device may be removed in a separate surgical procedure.

Recovery and Rehabilitation: Post-surgery, patients undergo intensive rehabilitation to regain strength, mobility, and function in the lengthened limb.

This phase is tailored to each individual's needs and may involve physical therapy, pain management, and ongoing monitoring for complications.

Limb lengthening surgery is a significant procedure that requires careful planning, skilled surgical intervention, and comprehensive post-operative care to achieve successful outcomes for patients seeking to address limb length discrepancies.

CHAPTER TWO

PREPARING FOR LIMB LENGTHENING SURGERY

Initial Consultation And Evaluations

The initial consultation for limb lengthening surgery is a crucial first step towards achieving your desired height or correcting limb deformities.

During this consultation, you will meet with your orthopedic surgeon to discuss your medical history, current condition, and goals for the surgery.

Expect a thorough evaluation of your limbs, including measurements and possibly imaging tests like X-rays or CT scans to assess bone structure and alignment. This evaluation helps the surgeon determine the feasibility and approach for the procedure tailored to your specific needs.

Psychological Preparation For Surgery

Preparing mentally for limb lengthening surgery is as important as physical preparation. This procedure can be challenging emotionally due to its length and the significant changes it brings.

It's normal to feel anxious or apprehensive. Psychological preparation involves understanding the surgery process, and potential outcomes, and discussing any concerns with your healthcare team. Consider seeking support from a counselor or support group to manage stress and maintain a positive mindset throughout the journey.

Physical Preparation And Pre-Operative Instructions

Physical preparation plays a crucial role in ensuring a smooth surgery and recovery process. Your surgeon will provide specific pre-operative instructions tailored to your case. This may include discontinuing certain medications, fasting before surgery, and maintaining a healthy lifestyle.

Follow these instructions closely to minimize risks and optimize your body's readiness for the procedure. Engage in light exercises as advised to maintain muscle strength and flexibility, which can aid in recovery post-surgery.

Anesthesia Options And Considerations

Anesthesia is a critical aspect of limb lengthening surgery. Your anesthesia options will be discussed during your pre-operative consultations.

Depending on the complexity of the surgery and your medical history, you may be offered general anesthesia, which renders you unconscious during the procedure, or regional anesthesia, which numbs only the surgical area while you remain awake.

Your anesthesiologist will review your health status and preferences to determine the safest and most effective anesthesia plan for you.

Preparing Your Home And Support System

Preparing your home environment and support system is essential for a successful recovery after limb-lengthening surgery.

Before the procedure, make necessary adjustments to your living space to accommodate potential mobility challenges.

This may include installing handrails, adjusting furniture heights, and ensuring clear pathways. Arrange for assistance from family members, friends, or professional caregivers during the initial recovery phase.

Having a supportive network in place can significantly ease your transition back home and enhance your overall recovery experience.

CHAPTER THREE

RECOVERY PHASE AND REHABILITATION

Immediate Post-Surgery Care

After limb lengthening surgery, immediate post-operative care is crucial for a successful recovery. You will likely wake up in a recovery room, where medical staff will closely monitor your vital signs and manage any immediate post-surgical pain or discomfort.

Pain management techniques may include medications prescribed by your surgeon to ensure you are as comfortable as possible during this initial phase.

Depending on the type of limb lengthening procedure you undergo—whether it's external fixation, internal lengthening nails, or other techniques—the specifics of your care may vary slightly.

External fixators, for example, require meticulous care to keep the pins and frames clean to prevent infections. Your surgical team will provide detailed instructions on how to care for these devices, including cleaning techniques and signs to watch for that may indicate a complication.

Managing Pain And Discomfort

Managing pain and discomfort following limb lengthening surgery is a top priority to ensure your comfort and support healing. Your medical team will prescribe pain medications tailored to your needs, which may include oral medications or, in some cases, intravenous pain relief immediately after surgery. It's essential to take these medications as directed to stay ahead of any potential pain.

Beyond medication, there are other strategies to manage discomfort effectively. Elevating the affected limb can help reduce swelling and discomfort while applying ice packs (if recommended by your surgeon) can also provide relief.

Maintaining a comfortable position in bed or while sitting is crucial, and your medical team will guide you on how to adjust positions safely.

Physical Therapy And Rehabilitation Exercises

Physical therapy and rehabilitation exercises play a pivotal role in the recovery process after limb lengthening surgery. Your physical therapist will create a personalized exercise plan designed to gradually restore strength, flexibility, and function to the affected limb.

These exercises typically begin once your surgeon clears you to start rehabilitation, usually within a few days to weeks post-surgery.

The initial focus of physical therapy may include gentle range of motion exercises and isometric muscle contractions to prevent stiffness and promote circulation. As you progress, your therapist will incorporate more challenging exercises to improve muscle strength and joint mobility. It's essential to follow your therapist's guidance closely and communicate any discomfort or concerns during sessions.

Nutritional Considerations For Recovery

Nutrition plays a critical role in supporting healing and recovery after limb-lengthening surgery. Your body requires increased nutrients, such as protein, vitamins, and minerals, to repair tissues and promote bone growth.

During the recovery phase, your healthcare team may recommend a balanced diet rich in lean proteins, fruits, vegetables, and whole grains to support optimal healing.

In some cases, your surgeon or a nutritionist may recommend specific supplements to ensure you're getting adequate nutrients.

These supplements may include calcium, vitamin D, or protein shakes to support bone health and overall recovery. Staying hydrated is also essential, as it helps maintain blood flow and supports cellular function during healing.

Monitoring Progress And Adjusting Treatment Plans

Throughout your recovery from limb lengthening surgery, regular monitoring of your progress is essential to ensure everything is healing as expected. Your surgeon will schedule follow-up appointments to assess the surgical site, monitor bone healing (if applicable), and evaluate your overall recovery. During these visits, they may perform X-rays or other imaging studies to track progress.

Based on these assessments, your treatment plan may be adjusted accordingly. This could involve modifying physical therapy exercises, adjusting pain management strategies, or providing additional medical interventions if complications arise.

Open communication with your healthcare team is crucial during this phase to address any concerns promptly and optimize your recovery outcome.

CHAPTER FOUR

POTENTIAL COMPLICATIONS AND RISKS

Common Complications During And After Surgery

Limb lengthening surgery, while transformative, involves certain risks that patients should be aware of. During the procedure, which typically includes the use of external fixators or internal devices, common complications can arise.

These may include infections around the surgical site, which are carefully monitored and treated promptly with antibiotics if detected.

Another potential issue is nerve or blood vessel damage, though this is rare and typically mitigated by the expertise of the surgical team.

After surgery, patients might experience pain, discomfort, or stiffness in the affected limb. This is normal as the body adjusts to the changes and begins the healing process.

Occasionally, there may be issues with the fixation devices, such as loosening or irritation at the pin sites. These are managed through regular check-ups and adjustments as needed by the orthopedic team.

Long-Term Risks And Challenges

While limb lengthening surgery offers significant benefits, long-term risks should be considered. Patients may face challenges such as uneven limb lengths, joint stiffness, or the need for additional surgeries to address residual issues.

The process of bone consolidation, where new bone forms and strengthens, is crucial but can sometimes lead to complications like delayed union or non-union of bones.

Over time, patients might also experience psychological effects related to their changed body image or lifestyle adjustments.

It's important for individuals undergoing this procedure to have realistic expectations and to follow post-operative care instructions diligently to minimize these risks.

Strategies For Complication Prevention

To mitigate risks during limb lengthening surgery, several strategies are employed. Pre-operative planning and thorough medical assessments ensure that patients are well-prepared for the procedure. Surgical techniques have advanced significantly, allowing for more precise corrections and reduced trauma to surrounding tissues. Post-operative care, including physical therapy and regular follow-ups, helps monitor progress and detect any potential complications early.

Addressing The Psychological Impact Of Surgery

The psychological impact of limb lengthening surgery can be profound. Patients may experience anxiety, depression, or body image concerns as they adjust to their changing appearance and capabilities.

Psychological support services, including counseling and support groups, are invaluable in helping individuals navigate these emotional challenges. Encouraging open communication between patients, families, and healthcare providers fosters a supportive environment where concerns can be addressed promptly.

Patient Stories And Coping Strategies

Many individuals who undergo limb lengthening surgery find strength in sharing their experiences and coping strategies. Hearing firsthand accounts from others who have walked a similar path can provide reassurance and practical tips for managing the recovery process.

Patients often highlight the importance of patience, persistence in physical therapy, and maintaining a positive mindset throughout their journey.

By learning from these narratives, individuals preparing for or recovering from surgery can feel more empowered and prepared for the road ahead.

CHAPTER FIVE

LIFE AFTER LIMB LENGTHENING SURGERY

Adjusting To New Limb Lengths

Adjusting to new limb lengths after limb lengthening surgery is a transformative process that involves both physical and psychological adaptation. Initially, patients may experience a range of sensations, from mild discomfort to a noticeable difference in gait and posture.

The adjustment period varies depending on individual factors such as the extent of lengthening and overall health.

Physically, as the bones gradually heal and new bone tissue forms, patients may need to use assistive devices like crutches or walkers to aid mobility. Physical therapy plays a crucial role in this phase, helping to strengthen muscles, improve flexibility, and regain functional movement patterns.

Therapists work closely with patients to develop personalized rehabilitation plans aimed at optimizing recovery and restoring normal daily activities.

Psychologically, adjusting to changes in limb length can be challenging. Patients may experience feelings of excitement, frustration, or anxiety as they adapt to their new physical appearance and capabilities. Patients need to receive support from healthcare professionals, family, and friends during this period to address emotional concerns and build confidence in their new body image.

Physical And Psychological Adaptation

Physical adaptation after limb lengthening surgery involves gradual changes as the bones heal and the body adjusts to the new length.

Patients typically experience improvements in mobility and function over time, supported by ongoing physical therapy and exercise routines.

Strengthening exercises focus on enhancing muscle tone and joint stability, aiding in the development of a balanced gait and posture.

Psychologically, adapting to the new limb length encompasses accepting and embracing the changes to body image and physical capabilities.

This process varies among individuals, influenced by factors such as pre-existing mental health, personal resilience, and social support systems.

Counseling and support groups can provide valuable emotional support, offering a platform for patients to share experiences and strategies for coping with the psychological aspects of recovery.

Returning To Daily Activities And Work

Returning to daily activities and work after limb lengthening surgery is a milestone that reflects both physical recovery and functional adaptation. As healing progresses, patients gradually resume activities of daily living, such as walking, climbing stairs, and performing household tasks.

Occupational therapists play a vital role in this phase, assessing functional abilities and recommending adaptations or modifications to facilitate a smooth transition back to daily routines.

Returning to work involves considerations such as ergonomic adjustments, gradual reintroduction of duties, and communication with employers regarding any necessary accommodations.

Patients may undergo vocational rehabilitation to ensure a successful return to their professional roles, supported by ongoing medical supervision to monitor healing and address any concerns that may arise.

Follow-Up Care And Monitoring

Follow-up care and monitoring are essential components of the post-operative phase following limb lengthening surgery. Regular appointments with orthopedic surgeons and rehabilitation specialists allow for ongoing assessment of healing progress, evaluation of functional outcomes, and adjustment of treatment plans as needed. Imaging studies, such as X-rays and bone scans, may be performed to monitor bone consolidation and detect any potential complications early.

Maintaining Long-term Bone Health

Maintaining long-term bone health is a lifelong commitment for individuals who have undergone limb-lengthening surgery. Adopting a balanced diet rich in calcium, vitamin D, and other essential nutrients supports bone strength and mineralization. Regular weight-bearing exercise, under the guidance of healthcare professionals, helps to preserve bone density and promote overall musculoskeletal health.

Monitoring bone health through periodic assessments, including bone density scans and blood tests, allows healthcare providers to identify and address any issues promptly. Patients are encouraged to adhere to recommended lifestyle modifications, such as avoiding smoking and excessive alcohol consumption, to minimize the risk of osteoporosis and other bone-related complications over time.

CHAPTER SIX

ALTERNATIVE TREATMENTS AND THERAPIES

Non-Surgical Options For Limb Length Discrepancies

When facing limb length discrepancies (LLDs), individuals often explore non-surgical options before considering more invasive treatments.

Non-surgical approaches primarily focus on managing symptoms and improving function without altering bone length. One common method is the use of orthotics, such as shoe lifts or custom-made shoe inserts.

These devices help balance the height differential between limbs, providing immediate relief and improved gait.

Physical therapy is another cornerstone of non-surgical management. Therapists design tailored exercise programs to strengthen muscles, improve flexibility, and correct posture.

By targeting specific muscle groups, physical therapy aims to optimize limb function and reduce discomfort associated with LLDs. Additionally, stretching exercises can help alleviate tightness in affected muscles, enhancing overall mobility and comfort.

For individuals with mild to moderate limb length differences, adaptive strategies in daily activities can be effective.

These strategies include adjusting seating positions, modifying workstations, and using assistive devices like canes or crutches to compensate for gait abnormalities.

These non-surgical approaches empower individuals to manage their condition proactively while maintaining functionality and comfort in daily life.

Comparative Benefits And Drawbacks

When considering treatments for limb length discrepancies (LLDs), weighing the benefits and drawbacks of each option is crucial.

Non-surgical interventions offer several advantages, including minimal invasiveness, lower risk of complications, and shorter recovery times compared to surgical procedures. They also provide immediate relief from symptoms such as pain and gait abnormalities, allowing individuals to maintain an active lifestyle without prolonged downtime.

However, non-surgical methods may have limitations, particularly in cases of significant LLDs where conservative measures alone may not achieve the desired outcomes.

Orthotic devices and physical therapy, while effective for many, may not address underlying skeletal discrepancies that require structural correction.

Furthermore, non-surgical approaches often necessitate ongoing management and adaptation, which can be cumbersome for some individuals.

In contrast, surgical interventions like limb lengthening procedures offer precise correction of bone length differentials, potentially improving overall limb symmetry and function. This approach is particularly beneficial for severe cases of LLDs where non-surgical methods have proven inadequate. Surgical techniques allow for targeted adjustments that can enhance both aesthetic appearance and functional capabilities, providing long-term benefits that non-surgical treatments may not achieve.

Integrative Therapies For Rehabilitation

Lifestyle Changes to Support Bone Health

Maintaining optimal bone health is essential for individuals undergoing rehabilitation following limb lengthening surgery. Adopting a bone-friendly lifestyle involves several key practices that promote bone strength and resilience. Adequate nutrition plays a critical role, emphasizing a diet rich in calcium, vitamin D, and other essential nutrients that support bone remodeling and healing. Foods such as dairy products, leafy greens, nuts, and fortified cereals are valuable sources of these nutrients.

Regular weight-bearing exercises are also vital for bone health. Activities such as walking, jogging, and weight training stimulate bone formation and density, helping to prevent osteoporosis and promoting healing after surgical interventions. Engaging in these exercises under the guidance of healthcare professionals ensures safety and effectiveness, tailored to individual rehabilitation needs and recovery stages.

In addition to dietary and exercise considerations, lifestyle adjustments may include smoking cessation and moderation of alcohol consumption, as these habits can negatively impact bone metabolism and healing processes. Maintaining a healthy body weight through balanced nutrition and regular physical activity further supports bone health, optimizing outcomes following limb lengthening surgery and enhancing overall well-being.

Case Studies And Patient Experiences

Understanding the real-life impact of limb-lengthening surgery through case studies and patient experiences provides valuable insights into treatment outcomes and recovery journeys.

Case studies often highlight individualized treatment plans, surgical techniques employed, and post-operative rehabilitation protocols tailored to each patient's unique needs and goals.

By examining these cases, healthcare providers and patients gain a comprehensive understanding of the complexities involved in managing limb length discrepancies.

Patient experiences offer firsthand perspectives on the emotional and physical aspects of undergoing limb-lengthening surgery.

These narratives often detail initial concerns, decision-making processes, surgical experiences, and recovery milestones.

By sharing their stories, patients contribute to a supportive community and offer encouragement to others considering similar treatments.

Patient testimonials also underscore the transformative impact of surgical interventions on quality of life, emphasizing resilience and optimism throughout the rehabilitation journey.

CHAPTER SEVEN

COMMON CONCERNS AND FAQS

Many individuals considering limb lengthening surgery often have several common concerns and questions. Addressing these upfront can help alleviate anxiety and provide clarity about the process.

One of the primary concerns is about the duration of the procedure. Limb lengthening surgery typically involves several stages, including the surgery itself and the subsequent lengthening phase. The entire process can take several months to over a year, depending on individual circumstances and the desired length increase.

Another frequently asked question revolves around the pain involved. Pain management is a crucial aspect of limb lengthening surgery. Patients are provided with various pain relief options, including medications and physical therapy, to ensure comfort throughout the recovery period.

Many patients also wonder about the risks associated with the surgery. While limb lengthening is generally safe when performed by experienced surgeons, like any surgical procedure, it carries risks such as infection, nerve damage, or complications related to the external fixator.

Addressing Pain Management Concerns

Effective pain management is essential for patients undergoing limb-lengthening surgery. The surgical team will discuss pain relief strategies before and after the procedure to ensure optimal comfort.

Immediately after surgery, pain medications are administered to control post-operative discomfort. These medications may include oral pain relievers and, in some cases, intravenous pain management for more intensive relief.

As the recovery progresses and the lengthening phase begins, the discomfort may shift to the area where the bones are being gradually extended. Pain management during this phase often involves a combination of pain medications tailored to the patient's needs, along with physical therapy to alleviate muscle stiffness and discomfort.

Dealing With Length Discrepancy Correction

Limb lengthening surgery aims to correct discrepancies in limb length caused by congenital conditions, injuries, or other medical issues. The process involves precise surgical techniques to lengthen the bone gradually.

During the initial consultation, the surgeon will assess the extent of the length difference and discuss the surgical approach.

The procedure typically involves making a precise cut in the bone (osteotomy) and gradually separating the bone segments using an external fixator or internal lengthening device.

The lengthening process itself is carefully monitored through regular appointments. Patients play an active role in their recovery by following prescribed lengthening protocols, which may include adjustments to the external fixator to gradually increase the length of the limb.

Managing External Fixator Or Device Discomfort

The external fixator or lengthening device used during limb lengthening surgery can initially feel uncomfortable or restrictive. Patients may experience sensations of tightness, pressure, or mild discomfort as they adjust to the device.

To manage discomfort, patients are provided with guidance on how to care for the fixator or device. This includes keeping the area clean and dry, adjusting the fixator as instructed by the surgeon, and performing gentle exercises to maintain mobility and reduce stiffness.

Psychological Support And Counseling Needs

Undergoing limb lengthening surgery can have significant psychological implications. Patients may experience emotions ranging from excitement about the potential outcome to anxiety or frustration during the recovery process.

Psychological support and counseling services are integral parts of comprehensive care. Patients are encouraged to discuss their feelings and concerns with a therapist or counselor who specializes in supporting individuals undergoing orthopedic procedures.

This support helps patients cope with the emotional aspects of surgery, manage expectations, and maintain a positive outlook throughout their recovery journey.

Guidance On Handling Post-Surgery Challenges

After limb lengthening surgery, patients may face various challenges as they progress through the lengthening and rehabilitation phases. These challenges can include physical discomfort, adjustments to daily activities, and emotional adjustments to the changes in their body.

Guidance on handling these challenges includes regular follow-up appointments with the surgical team to monitor progress, adjust the lengthening protocol as needed, and address any complications that may arise. Physical therapy plays a crucial role in restoring strength, flexibility, and function to the lengthened limb.

Patients are also advised on lifestyle modifications and self-care practices to promote healing and optimize recovery. This may include nutrition advice, proper wound care, and strategies to maintain mental and emotional well-being during the recovery process.

CHAPTER EIGHT

LOOKING AHEAD: ADVANCES IN LIMB LENGTHENING

Innovations In Surgical Techniques

Recent advancements in limb lengthening surgery have revolutionized treatment options for individuals seeking to correct limb length discrepancies or address congenital limb deformities. Traditional methods, such as the Ilizarov technique, have paved the way for newer, more sophisticated approaches that enhance both surgical precision and patient outcomes.

One notable innovation is the introduction of precise external fixation devices that allow for controlled distraction osteogenesis. These devices, often incorporating advanced computer-assisted technology, enable surgeons to accurately monitor and adjust the lengthening process throughout treatment. This method not only reduces the risk of complications but also promotes faster healing and improved functional outcomes for patients.

Moreover, minimally invasive techniques have gained popularity, offering reduced postoperative pain, shorter recovery times, and improved cosmetic results. Procedures like the PRECICE system utilize intramedullary nails that are remotely lengthened using an external magnetic mechanism, minimizing the need for external fixators and enhancing patient comfort during the lengthening phase.

Future Prospects For Limb-Lengthening Technology

Looking ahead, the future of limb-lengthening technology holds promising developments aimed at further improving patient experiences and outcomes. Researchers are exploring biocompatible materials and advanced biomaterial scaffolds that promote faster bone regeneration and integration. These materials not only support the bone-lengthening process but also reduce the risk of infections and complications associated with traditional methods.

Additionally, advancements in 3D printing technology are facilitating the customization of implants and external fixation devices tailored to individual patient anatomy. This personalized approach enhances surgical precision and promotes optimal bone healing, ultimately leading to better functional recovery and patient satisfaction.

The integration of robotics and artificial intelligence (AI) into limb-lengthening procedures is another exciting frontier. AI algorithms can analyze patient-specific data, predict optimal treatment plans, and assist surgeons in real time during complex surgical maneuvers. Robotics, on the other hand, offer unparalleled precision in bone cuts and fixation placement, further enhancing surgical outcomes and reducing recovery times.

Research And Development In Bone Regeneration

Bone regeneration therapies represent a burgeoning field in limb-lengthening research, aiming to accelerate healing and improve long-term bone integrity. Researchers are investigating the use of growth factors, stem cells, and tissue engineering techniques to stimulate bone formation and enhance the quality of newly formed tissue.

One promising approach involves the application of mesenchymal stem cells (MSCs) directly into the lengthened bone segment. These cells have the potential to differentiate into bone-forming cells and promote faster healing and integration of newly regenerated bone tissue.

Clinical trials are ongoing to evaluate the safety and efficacy of MSC-based therapies in enhancing bone regeneration outcomes in limb-lengthening procedures.

Furthermore, bioactive substances and scaffolds are being developed to create an optimal environment for bone growth and remodeling. These substances, when applied locally to the lengthened bone site, stimulate osteogenesis and angiogenesis, crucial processes for bone formation and vascularization. By enhancing the biological environment surrounding the lengthened bone, researchers aim to mitigate complications and expedite functional recovery for patients undergoing limb-lengthening surgery.

Patient Advocacy And Support Networks

Navigating limb-lengthening surgery can be emotionally and physically challenging for patients and their families. Patient advocacy groups and support networks play a crucial role in providing information, emotional support, and resources to individuals undergoing or considering limb-lengthening procedures.

These organizations offer educational materials, peer support forums, and access to experienced healthcare professionals who specialize in limb lengthening. By connecting patients with shared experiences and expert guidance, advocacy groups empower individuals to make informed decisions about their treatment journey and postoperative care.

Additionally, patient advocacy groups collaborate with healthcare providers and researchers to advocate for improved standards of care, accessibility to innovative treatments, and advancements in surgical techniques. By amplifying patient voices and promoting awareness, these networks contribute to the ongoing development and refinement of limb-lengthening practices worldwide.

Recommendations For Further Reading And Resources

For those interested in delving deeper into the field of limb-lengthening surgery, several authoritative resources provide comprehensive insights and research updates. Books such as "Limb Lengthening and Reconstruction Surgery" by Dr. S. Robert Rozbruch and Dr. Reggie C. Hamdy offer detailed explanations of surgical techniques, patient management strategies, and clinical outcomes in limb lengthening.

Medical journals such as the Journal of Limb Lengthening & Reconstruction and The Bone & Joint Journal frequently publish research articles, case studies, and reviews on advancements in limb-lengthening technology and bone regeneration therapies. These peer-reviewed publications serve as valuable resources for healthcare professionals, researchers, and students seeking to stay abreast of the latest developments in the field.

Furthermore, academic conferences and symposiums, such as the Annual Meeting of the Limb Lengthening and Reconstruction Society (LLRS), provide opportunities for networking, knowledge exchange, and continuing education in limb lengthening surgery. Attendees can engage with leading experts, participate in hands-on workshops, and explore innovative technologies shaping the future of orthopedic care.

By leveraging these resources and staying informed about ongoing research and clinical advancements, healthcare professionals and patients alike can contribute to the continued evolution and enhancement of limb-lengthening surgery outcomes.

www.ingramcontent.com/pod-product-compliance
Lightning Source LLC
Chambersburg PA
CBHW071844210526
45479CB00001B/274